AF875623

The Boob Chronicles: From Birth to Beyond

This version is intended to provide comprehensive information and support for breastfeeding mothers.

The Boob Chronicles: From Birth to Beyond

Table of Contents

Dedication

To my daughter, future children and breastfeeding moms!

Introduction to Breastfeeding

Breastfeeding is one of the most natural and intimate experiences a mother can share with her child. It not only provides essential nutrients that support the baby's growth and immune system, but it also fosters a deep, emotional bond that can last a lifetime. However, despite being a natural process, breastfeeding can come with challenges that require preparation, patience, and perseverance.

This guide aims to provide you with the knowledge and tools needed to navigate your breastfeeding journey successfully, whether you're a new mother or have previous experience.

What This Guide Covers

This guide will take you through every stage of breastfeeding, from the very first latch after birth to weaning your child when they are ready. We will cover practical tips, common challenges, and emotional aspects of breastfeeding. Additionally, you'll find advice on how to handle specific situations like breastfeeding after your baby grows teeth, dealing with biting, and the gradual process of weaning. Whether you plan to breastfeed for a few months or extend it for several years, this guide will serve as a reliable companion throughout your journey.

Benefits of Breastfeeding

Nutritional Benefits

Breast milk is uniquely tailored to meet your baby's nutritional needs. It contains the perfect balance of proteins, fats, vitamins, and minerals that are essential for healthy growth and development. Additionally, breast milk is packed with antibodies that help protect your baby from infections and illnesses. The composition of breast milk changes over time to meet the evolving needs of your baby, as compared to formula, which remains the same. Colostrum, the first milk produced after birth, is particularly rich in antibodies and nutrients that are crucial for your newborn's immune system.

Emotional and Psychological Benefits

The act of breastfeeding fosters a powerful emotional connection between the mother and child. The close physical contact, the warmth of your skin, and the soothing rhythm of your heartbeat create a sense of security and comfort for your baby. For mothers, breastfeeding releases oxytocin, a hormone that promotes feelings of love, bonding, and relaxation. This hormone also helps reduce stress levels, decreases the risk of postpartum depression, and enhances overall well-being. The emotional benefits of breastfeeding extend to both mother and child, creating a strong foundation for a lasting bond.

Long-Term Health Benefits

The benefits of breastfeeding extend far beyond infancy. For your baby, breastfeeding has been linked to a reduced risk of developing chronic conditions such as asthma, allergies, obesity, and Type 2 diabetes later in life. It also contributes to better cognitive development and a lower risk of Sudden Infant Death Syndrome (SIDS). For mothers, breastfeeding offers significant health benefits as well. It helps the uterus return to its pre-pregnancy size more quickly, reduces postpartum bleeding, and lowers the risk of breast and ovarian cancers. Additionally, breastfeeding can delay the return of menstruation, which may serve as a natural form of birth control during the early postpartum months.

Getting Started with Breastfeeding

Preparation During Pregnancy

Preparing for breastfeeding starts well before your baby arrives. During pregnancy, take the time to educate yourself about breastfeeding. This can include attending prenatal classes, reading books on breastfeeding, and discussing your breastfeeding goals with your healthcare provider. Understanding what to expect can help alleviate anxiety and increase your confidence. It's also helpful to have a support system in place, whether it's your partner, family members, or a lactation consultant, who can offer guidance and encouragement once your baby is born.

First Latch

The first latch is a pivotal moment in your breastfeeding journey. It is essential for establishing a healthy milk supply and ensuring that your baby is getting the nutrients they need. Immediately after birth, your baby is usually alert and ready to breastfeed. The first hour after birth, often referred to as the "golden hour," is the best time to initiate breastfeeding. During this time, place your baby skin-to-skin on your chest. This contact helps stimulate their natural instinct to latch onto your breast. Your baby may naturally nuzzle your breast and latch on when they are ready. If the latch is painful or if your baby seems to be struggling, seek assistance from a nurse or a lactation consultant.

Positioning

Proper positioning is key to a successful breastfeeding experience. A good latch is essential to prevent nipple pain and ensure that your baby is effectively extracting milk. There are several breastfeeding positions to choose from, including:

-***Cradle Hold:*** Your baby lies across your lap, facing you, with their head resting in the crook of your arm.

-***Cross-Cradle Hold:*** Similar to the cradle hold, with your opposite hand supporting your baby's head while the other hand supporting your breast.

-***Football Hold:*** Your baby is tucked under your arm like a football, with their body along your side and feet pointing toward your back.

-***Side-Lying Position:*** You and your baby lie on your sides facing each other. This position is especially helpful for nighttime feedings.

Experiment with these positions to find what works best for you and your baby. Ensure that your baby's mouth is wide open, with their lips flanged out like a fish, and their chin pressed against your breast. Their nose should be free, and they should take in a good portion of the areola, not just the nipple.

You will find examples on the next page on how to position the baby.

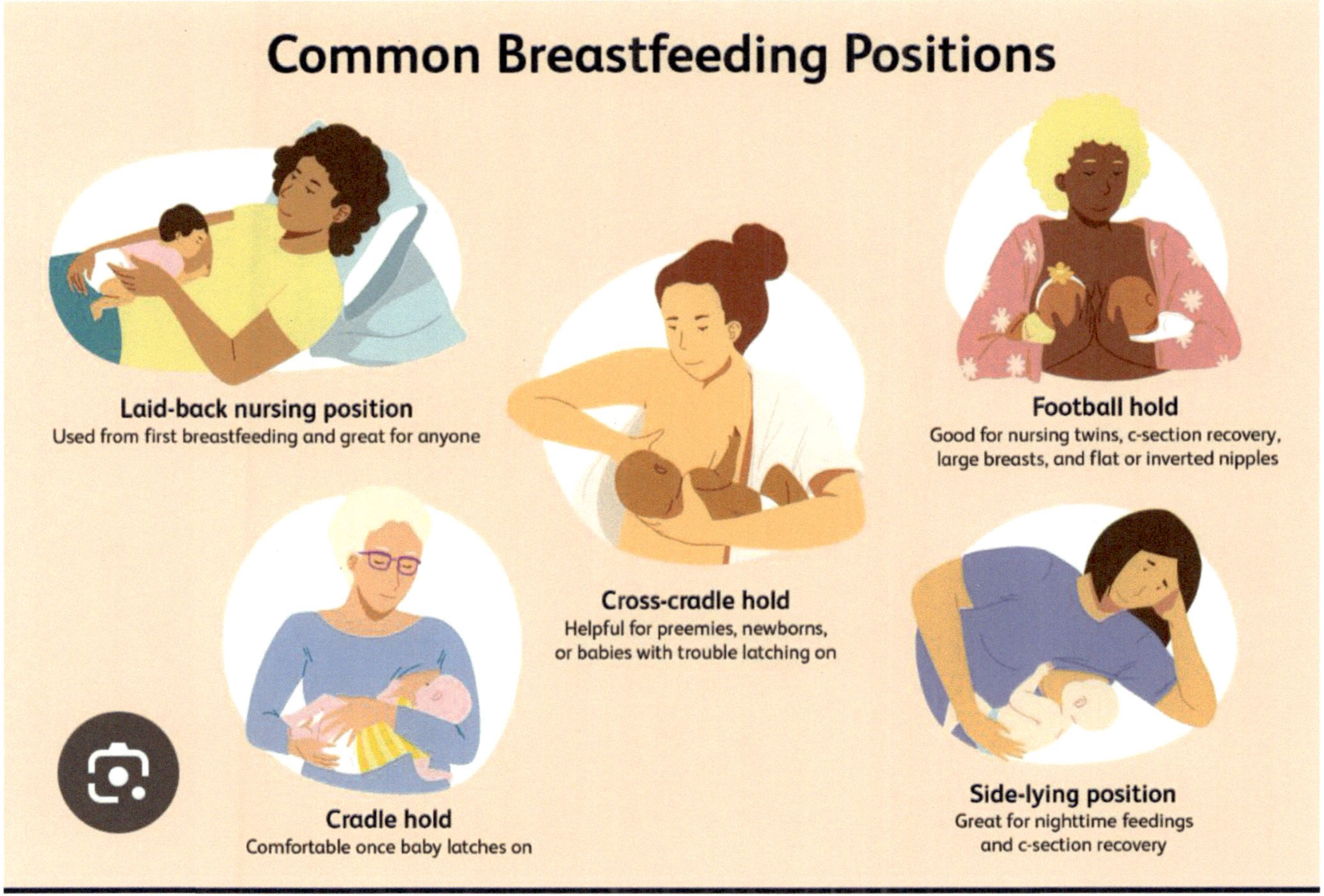
Common Breastfeeding Positions
Laid-back nursing position
Used from first breastfeeding and great for anyone
Cross-cradle hold
Helpful for preemies, newborns, or babies with trouble latching on
Football hold
Good for nursing twins, c-section recovery, large breasts, and flat or inverted nipples
Cradle hold
Comfortable once baby latches on
Side-lying position
Great for nighttime feedings and c-section recovery

Breastfeeding Challenges in the First Few Days

Common Issues

The first few days of breastfeeding can be overwhelming as both you and your baby learn together. Common issues include sore nipples, engorgement, and difficulties with latching. Sore nipples are often caused by an improper latch, so it's crucial to ensure your baby is latched on correctly. If soreness persists, try expressing a small amount of breast milk and applying it to your nipples to soothe them. Engorgement occurs when your breasts become overly full with milk, leading to swelling and discomfort. To alleviate engorgement, you can try nursing more frequently, using a warm compress before feeding, and expressing milk if necessary.

Another common issue is low milk supply, which can be concerning for many new mothers. However, frequent breastfeeding is the best way to stimulate milk production. Make sure your baby is feeding effectively, as a poor latch or infrequent nursing can impact your milk supply. If you are concerned about your milk supply, consult with a lactation consultant that can assess your breastfeeding technique and offer suggestions.

When to Seek Help

While many breastfeeding challenges can be resolved with proper technique and support, there are times when professional help is necessary. Seek assistance if:

- ***Breastfeeding is consistently painful.***

- Your baby isn't gaining weight or producing enough wet/dirty diapers.

- You notice symptoms of mastitis, such as breast redness, warmth, pain, and flu-like symptoms.

A lactation consultant can provide personalized advice and support to help you overcome these challenges. Don't hesitate to reach out for help—early intervention can prevent small issues from becoming bigger problems.

Establishing a Breastfeeding Routine

Feeding on Demand vs. Scheduled Feeding

One of the first decisions you'll need to make is whether to feed your baby on demand or follow a scheduled feeding routine. Feeding on demand means breastfeeding your baby whenever they show signs of hunger, such as rooting, sucking on their hands, or becoming fussy. Newborns typically need to eat every 1.5 to 3 hours, so feeding on demand can help establish your milk supply and ensure your baby is getting enough to eat.

Scheduled feeding, on the other hand, involves setting specific times for feeding. Some parents find this approach more predictable and easier to manage, especially if they have other children or responsibilities. However, it's important to remember that young babies often don't follow a strict schedule, so flexibility is key.

Ultimately, the choice between feeding on demand and scheduled feeding depends on your baby's needs and your lifestyle. Some mothers find that a combination of both works best. For example, you might feed on demand during the early weeks and gradually introduce a more predictable routine as your baby grows.

Nighttime Feedings

Nighttime feedings are an integral part of breastfeeding, especially during the first few months when your baby's stomach is still small, and they need to eat frequently. While nighttime feedings can be exhausting, they are crucial for maintaining your milk supply and ensuring your baby gets the calories they need to grow. From experience, the best time to nurse is between the hours of midnight and 4 am (12 am-4 am) for the most efficient supply and start of the day.

Creating a calm, dark environment can help make nighttime feedings more restful for both you and your baby. Consider room-sharing or co-sleeping (while following safe sleep guidelines) to make night feedings more convenient. If possible, try to catch up on sleep during the day by napping when your baby naps. Remember, frequent wake-ups won't last forever, and your baby will eventually start sleeping for longer stretches.

Nutrition and Diet for Breastfeeding Moms

Essential Nutrients

As a breastfeeding mother, your body needs extra nutrients to support milk production and maintain your health. A balanced diet rich in fruits, vegetables, whole grains, lean proteins, and healthy fats is essential. Some key nutrients to focus on include:

- ***Calcium:*** Found in dairy products, leafy greens, and fortified foods, calcium is vital for maintaining bone health.

- ***Iron:*** Lean meats, beans, and fortified cereals are good sources of iron, which helps prevent anemia.

- ***Omega-3 Fatty Acids:*** These healthy fats, found in fish like salmon and in flaxseeds, are important for your baby's brain development.

- ***Vitamin D:*** While it's difficult to get enough vitamin D from food alone, sunlight exposure and supplements can help ensure you're getting enough.

In addition to eating a nutritious diet, staying hydrated is crucial. Breastfeeding can make you feel thirsty, so drink plenty of water throughout the day. Keep a water bottle handy, especially during feedings.

Foods to Avoid or Limit

While most foods are safe to eat while breastfeeding, there are a few that should be consumed in moderation or avoided altogether. These include:

- ***Caffeine:*** While moderate caffeine consumption is generally safe, too much caffeine can make your baby irritable and disrupt their sleep. Limit your intake to 1-2 cups of coffee per day.

- ***Alcohol:*** If you choose to drink alcohol, wait at least 2-3 hours after consuming it before breastfeeding to allow the alcohol to metabolize.

- ***Certain Fish:*** Some fish, like shark, swordfish, and king mackerel, contain high levels of mercury, which can be harmful to your baby. Opt for low-mercury fish like salmon, tilapia, and shrimp.

- ***Allergenic Foods:*** If there is a history of food allergies in your family, you may want to be cautious about consuming common allergens like peanuts, tree nuts, and shellfish. However, most mothers can safely eat these foods unless their baby shows signs of an allergic reaction.

Breastfeeding After Baby Starts Growing Teeth

When Baby Starts Teething

Teething typically begins around 4-6 months of age, although it can start earlier or later (15-18 months) for some babies. As your baby's first teeth start to emerge, you may notice changes in their breastfeeding behavior. Some babies may nurse more frequently for comfort, while others may become fussier at the breast due to sore gums. You can help soothe your baby's discomfort by offering a cold teething ring or gently massaging their gums before feeding.

How to Handle Biting

One of the most common concerns for breastfeeding mothers is the possibility of their baby biting during feedings. While it can be painful, biting is usually a temporary phase that can be managed with a few strategies. When your baby bites, calmly remove them from the breast and firmly say "no." Avoid yelling or reacting strongly, as this can startle your baby. Offer them a teething toy to chew on instead, and then try breastfeeding again. Most babies will quickly learn that biting leads to the end of the feeding session.

If biting continues to be an issue, observe when it tends to happen. Babies are more likely to bite when they are teething, distracted, or are no longer hungry. Paying attention to your baby's cues can help you anticipate and prevent biting.

Breastfeeding with Teeth

It's entirely possible to continue breastfeeding after your baby has teeth. In fact, many mothers successfully breastfeed well into the toddler years without any issues. The key is to ensure that your baby maintains a proper latch. When latched correctly, your baby's tongue will cover their lower teeth, preventing them from biting. If you're concerned about breastfeeding with teeth, a lactation consultant can offer additional tips and reassurance.

Breastfeeding While Working

Planning for Your Return to Work

Returning to work doesn't mean you have to stop breastfeeding. With some planning and preparation, you can continue to provide your baby with breast milk even when you're not together. Before you return to work, start building a freezer stash of expressed milk by pumping once or twice a day. This will ensure you have plenty of milk to leave with your caregiver. Additionally, familiarize yourself with your workplace's breastfeeding policies and find out where you can pump during the day.

Pumping at Work

Pumping at work requires some logistical planning, but it's entirely doable. Aim to pump during the times your baby would normally nurse, which is usually every 3-4 hours. Invest in a high-quality double electric breast pump, which can help you express milk efficiently and comfortably. Make sure you have access to a private, clean space for pumping, and bring a cooler bag with ice packs to store your milk.

It's also helpful to have extra pump parts and storage bags on hand in case of emergencies. To make the pumping process more efficient, consider using a hands-free pumping bra so you can continue working while you pump. Don't forget to label and date your milk storage bags before refrigerating or freezing them.

Staying Connected with Your Baby

Even though you'll be apart from your baby during the workday, you can still maintain a strong breastfeeding relationship. Nurse your baby right before you leave for work and as soon as you return home. If possible, visit your baby during your lunch break to nurse. You can also ask your caregiver to bring your baby to your workplace for a mid-day feeding. Staying connected with your baby during the workday can help maintain your milk supply and provide comfort to both of you.

Pumping and Milk Storage

Choosing the Right Pump

Choosing the right breast pump is essential for successful pumping, especially if you plan to pump regularly. There are several types of pumps to choose from, including:

- ***Manual Pumps:*** These pumps are operated by hand and are best for occasional use.

- ***Single Electric Pumps:*** These pumps are powered by electricity and can express milk from one breast at a time.

- ***Double Electric Pumps:*** These pumps allow you to express milk from both breasts simultaneously, making them ideal for working mothers or those who need to pump frequently.

When selecting a pump, consider factors such as portability, noise level, suction strength, and ease of cleaning. Some insurance plans cover the cost of a breast pump, so be sure to check with your provider.

Pumping Techniques

Effective pumping involves finding a routine and technique that works for you. To maximize milk output, try to relax and create a comfortable environment for pumping. Looking at a photo or video of your baby, listening to soothing music, or using a warm compress on your breasts can help stimulate let-downs. Start with a low suction setting and gradually increase it to a comfortable level. Alternate between breasts every few minutes to encourage milk flow. If you're having trouble with let-down, try massaging your breasts or using breast compressions to help express more milk.

Milk Storage Guidelines

Proper storage of expressed breast milk is essential to ensure its safety and quality. Here are some general guidelines:

-Room Temperature: Freshly pumped milk can be stored at room temperature (77°F or colder) for up to 4 hours.

-Refrigerator: Store milk in the refrigerator at 39°F or colder for up to 4 days.

-Freezer: Milk can be stored in the freezer at 0°F or colder for up to 6 months. For longer storage, use a deep freezer where milk can last up to 12 months.

When storing milk, use BPA-free storage bags or containers specifically designed for breast milk. Label each container with the date and time the milk was expressed, and always use the oldest milk first. When thawing frozen milk, do so in the refrigerator overnight or by placing the container in warm water. Avoid using the microwave, as it can create hot spots and destroy valuable nutrients.

Breastfeeding Beyond Infancy

Extended Breastfeeding Benefits

Breastfeeding beyond infancy, also known as extended breastfeeding, offers numerous benefits for both mother and child. For toddlers, breast milk continues to provide valuable nutrients, antibodies, and comfort. Extended breastfeeding has been linked to better immune function, higher IQ scores, and stronger social-emotional development. For mothers, extended breastfeeding can offer continued health benefits, such as reduced risk of certain cancers and osteoporosis.

Social and Cultural Considerations

In some cultures, extended breastfeeding is the norm, while in others, it may be less common and even discouraged. It's important to remember that breastfeeding is a personal decision, and there is no "right" time to wean. You may encounter opinions from family, friends, or even healthcare providers, but ultimately, the decision should be based on what feels right for you and your child. Surround yourself with supportive individuals who respect your choice to continue breastfeeding as long as you and your child desire.

Balancing Breastfeeding with Solid Foods

As your baby approaches their first birthday, solid foods will become an increasingly important part of their diet. However, breast milk should still be a significant source of nutrition. You may notice that your toddler starts to nurse less frequently as they eat more solid foods, but this doesn't mean breastfeeding should be discontinued. Continue to offer the breast before or after meals, depending on your child's preference. Breastfeeding can complement a healthy diet of solid foods, providing essential nutrients and comfort during this transitional stage.

Breastfeeding and Maternal Health

Physical Recovery Postpartum

Breastfeeding plays a vital role in your postpartum recovery. The act of breastfeeding triggers the release of oxytocin, a hormone that helps your uterus contract and return to its pre-pregnancy size. This process reduces postpartum bleeding and promotes faster recovery. Additionally, breastfeeding helps burn extra calories, which can aid in weight loss after pregnancy. However, it's important to remember that every woman's body is different, and weight loss may vary.

Mental and Emotional Well-being

Breastfeeding has a positive impact on your mental and emotional well-being. The release of oxytocin during breastfeeding promotes relaxation and reduces stress levels. This hormone also helps lower the risk of postpartum depression by enhancing feelings of bonding and contentment. However, breastfeeding can sometimes feel overwhelming, especially if you encounter challenges. It's essential to prioritize self-care and seek support from loved ones or professionals if needed. Remember that taking care of your mental health is just as important as your physical health.

Breastfeeding and Exercise

Many mothers wonder when it's safe to resume exercise after giving birth. Generally, you can start with light activities like walking as soon as you feel ready. More intense exercise can usually be resumed after your postpartum check-up, typically around six weeks after birth. Breastfeeding and exercise can coexist without negatively impacting your milk supply as long as you stay hydrated and listen to your body. If you're concerned about your milk supply, consider nursing your baby before exercising or expressing milk beforehand.

Breastfeeding During Illness

When You're Sick

If you come down with a common illness like a cold or the flu, it's usually safe to continue breastfeeding. In fact, breastfeeding can help protect your baby from getting sick, as your body produces antibodies that are passed through your milk. It's important to rest, stay hydrated, and continue nursing as usual. If you're taking medication, consult your healthcare provider to ensure it's safe for breastfeeding. Most over-the-counter medications are compatible with breastfeeding, but some may need to be avoided.

When Baby is Sick

Breastfeeding is one of the best ways to comfort and nourish your baby when they're sick. Breast milk is easy to digest and provides hydration, nutrients, and antibodies that can help your baby recover more quickly. Your baby may nurse more frequently when they're not feeling well, as breastfeeding provides comfort and relief. It's also normal for sick babies to nurse for shorter periods or be fussier at the breast. Follow your baby's lead, and offer the breast frequently to ensure they're getting enough fluids.

Weaning: When and How to Start

Signs It's Time to Wean

Weaning is a gradual process that happens at a different pace for every mother and child. Some signs that it may be time to start weaning include your baby showing less interest in breastfeeding, eating more solid foods, or naturally reducing the number of nursing sessions. You might also feel ready to stop breastfeeding due to personal reasons, such as returning to work, a new pregnancy, or simply feeling that it's the right time.

Gradual Weaning Process

Weaning doesn't have to be an all-or-nothing process. Gradual weaning allows your baby to adjust to the change while minimizing discomfort for you. Start by eliminating one nursing session at a time, beginning with the session your baby is least interested in. Replace the feeding with a cup of milk or a healthy snack. After a few days or weeks, drop another session. Continue this process until your baby is fully weaned. If your baby resists weaning, try offering extra cuddles and comfort for an easy transition.

Emotional Aspects of Weaning

Weaning can be an emotional experience for both you and your baby. It's natural to feel a sense of loss or sadness as this special phase comes to an end. However, it's also an opportunity to celebrate the bond you've shared and the milestones you've achieved together. Be patient with yourself and your baby during this transition, and remember that weaning doesn't mean the end of your connection—it simply marks the beginning of a new chapter.

Breastfeeding in Special Situations

Tandem Nursing

Tandem nursing refers to breastfeeding two children of different ages, such as a toddler and a newborn, at the same time. This situation often arises when a mother continues to breastfeed an older child during a subsequent pregnancy. Tandem nursing can be a rewarding experience, allowing you to maintain your bond with both children. It's important to ensure that your newborn gets priority at the breast to establish your milk supply and meet their nutritional needs. Your body will continue to produce enough milk for both children, but their needs and feeding patterns may differ.

Breastfeeding Multiples

Breastfeeding multiples, such as twins or triplets, presents unique challenges, but it's entirely possible with the right support and strategies. The key to success is establishing a routine that works for you and your babies. Consider feeding both babies simultaneously using positions like the football hold or a twin nursing pillow. This approach can save time and ensure that both babies are fed adequately. Pumping can also be helpful if one baby is having difficulty latching or if you need to supplement with expressed milk. Seeking support from a lactation consultant experienced with multiples can provide valuable guidance.

Breastfeeding After Surgery

Breastfeeding after surgery, whether it's a cesarean section or another type of surgery, may require some adjustments but is generally safe and possible. If you've had a cesarean section, finding a comfortable breastfeeding position that doesn't put pressure on your incision is crucial. The side-lying or football-holding positions are often recommended. If you're taking pain medication or other medications after surgery, consult your healthcare provider to ensure they're safe for breastfeeding. In most cases, breastfeeding-compatible options are available.

Breastfeeding Myths and Facts

Myth: Breastfeeding Hurts

One of the most common misconceptions about breastfeeding is that it's supposed to hurt. While some discomfort during the first few days is normal as your body adjusts, ongoing pain is not. Persistent pain is often a sign of an improper latch or another issue that needs to be addressed. A proper latch should feel comfortable, and your baby should be able to nurse without causing pain. If you're experiencing pain, seek help from a lactation consultant who can evaluate your technique and offer solutions.

Fact: You Can Breastfeed After Returning to Work

Many mothers believe that returning to work means they have to stop breastfeeding, but this is not the case. With the right planning and support, you can continue to breastfeed after returning to work. Pumping during the day allows you to maintain your milk supply and provide breast milk for your baby while you're apart. Many workplaces offer accommodations for breastfeeding mothers, such as designated pumping spaces and flexible schedules. Communicate your needs with your employer to ensure you have the support you need to continue breastfeeding.

Myth: You Can't Breastfeed with Small Breasts

Breast size has no impact on your ability to breastfeed. Breast milk production is determined by the demand for milk, not the size of your breasts. Women with small breasts can produce just as much milk as women with larger breasts. The key to successful breastfeeding is ensuring that your baby is nursing effectively and frequently. If you're concerned about your milk supply, focus on proper latching techniques, frequent nursing, and staying hydrated.

Self-Care for Breastfeeding Moms

The Importance of Self-Care

Breastfeeding can be demanding, both physically and emotionally, so it's essential to prioritize self-care. Taking care of yourself not only benefits you but also ensures that you have the energy and well-being to care for your baby. Self-care can include a variety of activities, such as taking short breaks to rest, enjoying a warm bath, practicing mindfulness or meditation, and engaging in gentle exercises like yoga. It's also important to seek support from your partner, family, or friends so you don't feel overwhelmed.

Managing Stress

Stress can impact your milk supply and overall well-being, so finding ways to manage stress is crucial. Identify the sources of stress in your life and consider ways to reduce or eliminate them. This might involve delegating tasks, setting boundaries, or seeking help from others. Mindfulness practices, such as deep breathing exercises and meditation, can help you stay calm and centered during challenging moments. Additionally, connecting with other breastfeeding mothers through support groups or online communities can provide valuable encouragement and reduce feelings of isolation.

Finding Time for Yourself

Finding time for yourself can be challenging when you're caring for a newborn, but it's important to carve out moments for self-care. Whether it's a few minutes to enjoy a cup of tea, read a book, or take a short walk, these small breaks can help recharge your energy and boost your mood. Don't hesitate to ask for help from your partner or loved ones so you can have some time to yourself. Remember, taking care of yourself is not selfish—it's essential for your well-being and your ability to care for your baby.

Building a Breastfeeding Support System

The Role of Your Partner

Your partner plays a crucial role in your breastfeeding journey. Their support and encouragement can make a significant difference in your experience. Encourage your partner to be involved in the breastfeeding process by helping with tasks like bringing the baby to you for feedings, burping the baby afterward, or preparing snacks and drinks for you while you nurse. Open communication is key—discuss your breastfeeding goals and any challenges you're facing so your partner can offer the support you need.

Family and Friends

Family and friends can also be valuable sources of support during your breastfeeding journey. Don't hesitate to reach out to them for help with household tasks, childcare for older siblings, or simply to provide a listening ear. Educating your loved ones about breastfeeding can help them understand the challenges you may face and the importance of their support. Some mothers find it helpful to join a breastfeeding support group where they can connect with other mothers who are going through similar experiences.

Professional Support

Lactation consultants are trained professionals who specialize in breastfeeding support. They can provide personalized advice, troubleshoot problems, and offer encouragement during difficult times. Many hospitals and birthing centers have lactation consultants on staff who can assist you after delivery. If you're experiencing ongoing challenges, consider scheduling a one-on-one consultation with a lactation consultant who can observe a feeding session and provide tailored guidance. Additionally, some insurance plans cover lactation consultations, so be sure to check your coverage.

Breastfeeding Around the World

Cultural Practices

Breastfeeding practices vary widely around the world, influenced by cultural beliefs, traditions, and social norms. In some cultures, breastfeeding is seen as the natural and expected way to feed a baby, with extended breastfeeding being the norm. In other cultures, formula feeding may be more common, or breastfeeding in public may be less accepted. Understanding the cultural context of breastfeeding can help you navigate your own breastfeeding journey and respect the choices of others.

Global Breastfeeding Initiatives

Several global initiatives promote and support breastfeeding as a vital public health strategy. The World Health Organization (WHO) and UNICEF recommend exclusive breastfeeding for the first six months of life, followed by continued breastfeeding along with complementary foods for up to two years or beyond. The Baby-Friendly Hospital Initiative (BFHI) is one such program that encourages hospitals and birthing centers to adopt practices that support breastfeeding. Additionally, World Breastfeeding Week, celebrated annually from August 25-31, raises awareness about the importance of breastfeeding and promotes breastfeeding-friendly policies worldwide.

Lessons from Around the World

Different countries offer valuable lessons on how to create a supportive environment for breastfeeding mothers. For example, in Norway, generous maternity leave policies and widespread public acceptance of breastfeeding have contributed to high breastfeeding rates. In contrast, countries with shorter maternity leave and less social support may have lower breastfeeding rates. Learning from these global examples can inspire efforts to improve breastfeeding support in your own community.

Resources for Breastfeeding Moms

Online Resources

The internet offers a wealth of resources for breastfeeding mothers, from informative websites to supportive online communities. Some reputable websites include:

-La Leche League International: A global organization that provides breastfeeding information and support through articles, forums, and local support groups.

-KellyMom: A comprehensive resource for breastfeeding, parenting, and maternal health, offering evidence-based information on a wide range of topics.

-Breastfeeding USA: A nonprofit organization that provides breastfeeding support through peer counselors, articles, and a community forum.

Books and Literature

Books can be an excellent source of information and inspiration during your breastfeeding journey. Some recommended titles include:

-"The Womanly Art of Breastfeeding" by La Leche League International: A classic guide that covers all aspects of breastfeeding, from newborn nursing to weaning.

-"Breastfeeding Made Simple" by Nancy Mohrbacher and Kathleen Kendall-Tackett: A practical guide that offers step-by-step advice for overcoming common breastfeeding challenges.

- "The Nursing Mother's Companion" by Kathleen Huggins: A comprehensive reference book that provides detailed information on breastfeeding, including troubleshooting tips and solutions for various issues.

Support Groups

Joining a support group can provide you with a sense of community and connection with other breastfeeding mothers. Many hospitals, birthing centers, and community organizations offer breastfeeding support groups where you can share experiences, ask questions, and receive encouragement. Online support groups and forums are also available for mothers who prefer virtual connections. Some popular online support groups include:

-La Leche League Facebook Groups: These groups offer peer support and information for mothers at all stages of breastfeeding.

-Breastfeeding Support on Reddit: An active online community where mothers can ask questions, share experiences, and receive advice from other breastfeeding mothers.

-The Bump Breastfeeding Forum: A forum where mothers can connect with others and discuss breastfeeding topics in a supportive environment.

Conclusion

Celebrating Your Breastfeeding Journey

Breastfeeding is a unique and deeply personal experience that requires dedication, patience, and love. Whether you breastfeed for a few weeks, a few months, or a few years, each moment is an opportunity to nourish and bond with your baby. It's important to celebrate your achievements, no matter how big or small, and to recognize the incredible effort you've put into providing the best start for your child.

Embracing Flexibility

Every breastfeeding journey is different, and it's okay if things don't go exactly as planned. Embrace flexibility and be gentle with yourself as you navigate the ups and downs of breastfeeding. Remember that there is no "perfect" way to breastfeed—what matters most is that you and your baby are healthy, happy, and connected.

Looking to the Future

As you move forward in your breastfeeding journey, continue to seek out support, information, and encouragement. The knowledge and experience you've gained will serve you well, whether you're planning to breastfeed another child in the future or simply want to support other mothers on their breastfeeding journeys. Remember, you're not alone—millions of mothers around the world are sharing this journey with you, and together, you're creating a brighter, healthier future for the next generation.

This 20-page guide is designed to provide comprehensive, practical information to support mothers on their breastfeeding journey. From the early days of nursing to navigating challenges like teething and returning to work, this guide covers a wide range of topics to help mothers feel confident and empowered. The guide also emphasizes the importance of self-care, support systems, and embracing the unique aspects of each breastfeeding experience. Whether you're a first-time mom or a seasoned breastfeeding veteran, this guide offers valuable insights and encouragement to help you succeed in your breastfeeding goals.

About the Author

Chelsea D. Thoby is an island gyal with deep roots in the Bahamas and Barbados, raised amidst the vibrant culture of Miami. As a proud first-generation college graduate on her mother's side, Chelsea exemplifies determination and resilience. She earned her undergraduate degree in Biology from the illustrious Florida Agricultural and Mechanical University (FAMU) in Tallahassee, Florida, and furthered her education with a Master's degree in Public Health from Purdue University Global.

Balancing multiple roles, Chelsea is a devoted new mom to a beautiful 17-month-old baby girl, a loving wife, and a caring sister, aunt, and friend. Her nurturing spirit extends beyond her family as she also serves as a doula, supporting other mothers in their journeys. In addition to her human family, Chelsea is a dedicated dog mom, embracing the joy and companionship her furry friend brings into her life.

Chelsea's story is one of perseverance, love, and commitment to both her family and her professional aspirations, reflecting the strength of her heritage and the values instilled in her upbringing.

Made in the USA
Monee, IL
05 November 2026

67385755R00029